Cycling and Energy Snacking

Optimal Fuel for Your Journey

Table of Contents

Chapter 1. Introduction

Unlock the unlimited potential of your two-wheeled adventures with our expertly-crafted Special Report on 'Cycling and Energy Snacking: Optimal Fuel for Your Journey'. Deep dive into the science of sustained energy, on and off-road nutrition strategies, and uncover the power of well-timed snacking. Whether you're gearing up for your next grand tour, or simply cycling home from work, knowing the best fuel for your journey can drastically improve your performance and overall experience. Delivered in an easily digestible format, this dynamic guide blends practical advice with fascinating insights. Our special report is your ticket to healthier, more effective cycling sessions. So, gear up and prepare to pedal your way through this illuminating guide. Let's make your next ride, your best ride!

Chapter 2. The Physiology of Cycling and Metabolic Demands

A leisurely cycling session, a grueling hill climb, or an adrenaline-pumping race, each of the cycling variations involves its own complexity and strain on the human body. To fully comprehend how one can optimize energy snacking during cycling, it's crucial to understand the underlying physiology of cycling and the metabolic demands it imposes on the body.

2.1. The Biomechanics of Cycling

Cycling, while being a common mode of transportation and a popular pastime, is also a distinct biomechanical process that engages various muscle groups. Primarily, it involves the quadriceps, hamstrings, gluteal muscles, and calf muscles.

Typically, the downstroke phase, the 'activation phase,' involves primarily the quadriceps and gluteal muscles. Conversely, the upstroke phase, or the 'recovery phase,' involves the hamstring and calf muscles. This constant interplay of muscle groups suggests cycling is a lower body-intensive activity, placing significant metabolic demands on these muscle collections.

2.2. Energy System Involved in Cycling

Cycling is an aerobic sport, which means it mainly depends on the aerobic energy system, also known as the oxygen system. However, other energy systems – the ATP-PC (adenosine triphosphate -

phosphocreatine) system and the Anaerobic Glycolysis system—play crucial roles depending on the intensity and duration of cycling.

When you start cycling, the body initially relies on the ATP-PC system for quick bursts of energy, which generally lasts around 10 to 15 seconds. As the activity continues, the anaerobic glycolysis system kicks in, breaking down glucose without oxygen to create energy, resulting in by-products like lactate. This system can fuel the body for up to a minute at high intensity.

Following that, the body reverts to the aerobic system for sustainable and long-term energy production. The aerobic system utilizes oxygen to break down glucose, producing a considerable amount of energy with water and carbon dioxide as by-products.

2.3. Metabolic Considerations During Cycling

The body's capability to meet energy demands during cycling is influenced by two significant metabolic considerations - VO2 max and the lactate threshold.

VO2 max, or maximal oxygen uptake, is a determinant of a cyclist's cardiorespiratory fitness level. It refers to the maximum amount of oxygen the body can utilize during intensive exercise. The higher the VO2 max, the better the cardiovascular fitness, allowing longer durations of cycling before fatigue sets in.

The Lactate threshold, on the other hand, is the point at which lactic acid (or lactate) starts to accumulate in the muscles during high-intensity cycling. Crossing this threshold leads to rapid fatigue and a decrease in performance. Through training, however, the lactate threshold can be improved, permitting higher intensity riding for longer periods.

2.4. Nutrition and Metabolic Demand

Cycling, characterized by long durations and varying intensity levels, requires a balanced approach to nutrition to meet its metabolic demands.

Carbohydrates are the predominant energy source during cycling, primarily supplying the aerobic energy system. Therefore, cyclists should prioritize complex carbohydrate intake for sustained energy release.

Fat also serves as a significant energy source during lower-intensity, longer duration rides. A well-trained athlete can tap into their fat stores efficiently, saving glycogen stores for more intense periods of cycling.

Protein doesn't significantly contribute to energy during cycling but is vital during the recovery phase for repairing and building muscle tissue.

Ensuring appropriate micronutrient intake, like vitamins and minerals, is additionally essential for optimal metabolic functioning and maintaining a robust immune system.

Understanding the demands of cycling on the human body and the metabolic requirements can guide the development of a thoughtfully planned energy snacking strategy. The subsequent sections will delve deeper into the art and science of energy snacking and its pivotal role in optimizing your cycling journey.

Chapter 3. Understanding Energy Sources: Fats, Carbs and Proteins

To optimally fuel physical activities, particularly endurance sports such as cycling, understanding the different energy sources – mainly fats, carbohydrates, and proteins – is crucial. Understanding these macronutrients help provide insights on the body's energy utilization processes, dietary and snacking strategies for the cycling journey and their impact on the cyclist's performance.

3.1. Understanding Carbohydrates

Carbohydrates are the body's preferred source of fuel during high-intensity activities. They provide immediate energy and are central to muscle contractions. Once consumed, the body breaks down carbohydrates into glucose molecules, which feed the body's cells. During high-intensity cycling, the body primarily utilizes glucose stored in the muscles and liver as glycogen.

There are two main types of carbohydrates: simple and complex. Simple carbohydrates, found in fruits, milk, and added sugars, provide a quick burst of energy due to their easy-to-digest nature. Complex carbohydrates, on the other hand, found in whole grains, legumes, vegetables, are slowly digested, providing a more steady release of energy.

Eating a carbohydrate-rich diet prior to cycling can enhance muscular glycogen stores. However, considering that glycogen stores are finite, strategies for replenishing these resources during extended cycling sessions should be examined. This is where cycling snacks or energy gels high in carbohydrates come into play.

3.2. Understanding Fats

While carbohydrates supply immediate and short-term energy, fats serve as a long-lasting fuel source. Contrary to common misconceptions, fat is not an enemy, particularly for endurance athletes. Stored body fat can provide a massive energy reserve - a typical lean adult stores enough body fat to fuel weeks of continuous exercise.

Fat, which gets broken down into fatty acids and glycerol through the process of lipolysis, is metabolized rather slowly. As such, it provides energy over a longer duration and is primarily utilized during low to moderate-intensity activity, or once carbohydrate stores have been depleted.

It is important to include fats as part of the healthy cyclist's diet, focusing on unsaturated fats from sources such as avocados, fatty fish, nuts, seeds, and olive oil. However, during the actual cycling event or intense workout, the focus should remain primarily on carbohydrates due to their quicker accessibility.

3.3. Understanding Proteins

Proteins are the building blocks of the body, crucial for muscle recovery and development, but are less frequently used as a source of energy. Protein consists of amino acids, nine of which are essential and must be sourced from the food we consume.

While typically not a significant energy source during shorter rides, proteins may contribute to 5-15% of the energy expenditure in endurance events. However, protein's most critical contribution for cyclists comes post-ride. Consuming protein after cycling promotes recovery by repairing muscle tissue and promoting muscle growth.

Intake of some amount of protein in snacks during long, strenuous rides (2-3 hours or more) can help mitigate muscle damage. But it's essential to balance protein with enough carbohydrates to maintain energy levels.

3.4. Balancing Energy Sources

A balanced and varied diet that includes carbohydrates, fats, and proteins is crucial for both performance and health. In meals, a cyclist should aim to fill half the plate with high-fiber foods rich in carbohydrates (like fruits, vegetables, and whole grains), a quarter with lean proteins (like fish, lean meats, or legumes), and the remaining quarter with unsaturated fats.

Pre-ride meals, consumed 2-4 hours before cycling, should majorly focus on carbohydrates, with some protein. Meanwhile, for post-ride, the emphasis should shift towards proteins (to aid muscle recovery), again, not forgetting carbohydrates to replenish glycogen stores.

3.5. Snacking Effectively: The Timing and Quantity

To further understand how to best employ these nutrients, let's talk about patterns of consumption. During extended periods of cycling, carbohydrate stores (glycogen) start to run low. Consuming carbohydrate-rich snacks, like energy bars or gels during the ride, can help maintain energy levels and prevent fatigue.

If cycling for an hour or less, there's typically no need for any in-ride nutrition. For rides of 1-3 hours, try to consume around 30-60g of carbohydrates each hour. For rides over 3 hours, aim for around 60-90g of carbohydrates per hour.

Integrating fat and protein into your performance diet can be bit intricate. Fat, as a slower-metabolized energy source, can fuel longer, less-intense workouts. Consuming a meal rich in healthy fats hours before a ride can provide sustained energy. Protein consumption helps rebuild and repair muscles post-ride, although some protein can be beneficial during long rides to prevent muscle breakdown.

Note that the above metrics can vary based on your body weight, the intensity of the cycling, and your overall nutritional needs. It is always beneficial to seek advice from a nutritionist or dietitian who specializes in sports nutrition to precisely plan your dietary and snacking strategies.

Understanding and leveraging the right macronutrients in the proper amounts at the right time are integral for an efficient and strong ride. The science of fueling isn't just about what you eat, but when and how you consume it, making knowledge your most powerful tool in creating a nutrition strategy that suits your unique needs. Happy cycling!

Chapter 4. Burning Calories: The Need for Fuel During a Ride

Understanding how the body utilizes energy during cycling is crucial for efficiently fueling your rides and improving your performance. This section delves into the science of calorie burning and the importance of well-timed, nutrient-dense snacking for sustaining your power throughout the ride.

4.1. The Human Power Plant

At its very core, the human body is akin to a sophisticated machine or power plant. However, unlike a maintenance-free power plant, the body produces energy from food that it converts into fuel. It then uses this fuel to perform every function—from breathing and digestion, to intense physical activity such as cycling.

The food we consume is broken down into macronutrients: carbohydrates, proteins, and fats. Each of these serves a specific purpose in fueling your body, and understanding their roles can help optimize your nutrition for cycling.

1. **Carbohydrates:** Often considered the body's primary energy source, carbohydrates are converted into glucose, which fuels your muscles and brain. During high-intensity activities, such as cycling, the body relies heavily on carbohydrates to maintain performance.

2. **Proteins:** While not the body's first choice for energy, proteins are essential for muscle repair and recovery after intense exercise. Amino acids, the building blocks of proteins, aid in the repair of muscle tissues that can be damaged during rigorous

cycling sessions.

3. **Fats:** As the most energy-dense macronutrient, fat provides over twice as much energy per gram as carbohydrates or proteins. However, it's a slower, less efficient energy source. During low to moderate intensity exercise, the body draws upon fat stores for energy.

4.2. The Caloric Balance in Cycling

For many cyclists, understanding the caloric balance—how many calories are consumed versus how many are burned—is key to managing energy levels and performance. While energy needs will vary based on factors such as ride duration, intensity, individual metabolism, and body size, a general rule of thumb is that the average cyclist burns approximately 400 to 500 calories per hour.

To fuel adequately, it's recommended that cyclists ingest about 30 to 60 grams of carbohydrates per hour during long rides, which roughly translates to 120-240 calories. Keep in mind that the body can only process a limited amount of carbohydrates at a time, so the upper limit is typically around 60 grams per hour.

Remember that while burning calories is a natural part of cycling, the goal shouldn't be to burn as many as possible. Instead, aim to maintain a balance that supports your energy needs, promotes recovery, and sustains overall health. In other words, calories aren't necessarily your enemy but rather a measure of energy that should be used smartly to fuel your ride.

4.3. On-the-go Nutritional Strategies

During a ride, regular snacking can help replenish your depleting energy levels, reduce fatigue, and maintain overall performance. Timing is paramount—you should aim to consume your first snack 30-60 minutes into your ride and then refuel every 15-30 minutes thereafter. But what should these snacks consist of?

- Easily Digested Carbohydrates: As your body quickly uses up stored glucose (aka glycogen), it's vital to refuel with easily digestible carbs. Energy gels, bars, and certain fruits, such as bananas or dates, are performance favourites.

- Hydration Plus Electrolytes: Thirst isn't the best measure of hydration status, so regular, even sipping of water is recommended. Including electrolytes in your hydration strategy can help replace the salts lost through sweat and maintain fluid balance.

- A Small Dose of Protein: During prolonged exercises, having a small source of protein can help ward off muscle damage. Keep in mind, though, that protein can be more difficult for the body to break down and digest during a ride, so it should not comprise the main component of on-the-go snacks.

While these are generally reliable strategies, it's important to test different nutrition approaches to find what works best for your body and for different ride conditions.

4.4. Post-Ride Refueling

After your ride, your body is in a state of repair. Consuming a balanced mix of carbohydrates and protein in a 3:1 or 4:1 ratio is recommended to replenish lost glycogen stores and promote muscle recovery. The body is most receptive to restoring glycogen stores within the first 30 minutes to two hours post-ride, so don't delay your meal. Options might include a chicken or tuna sandwich, a bowl of pasta with lean protein, yogurt with fruits and nuts, or a simple protein shake with a piece of fruit.

By understanding how your body burns energy and using this knowledge to fuel your rides effectively, you can unlock the true potential of your cycling performance. Remember, good fueling isn't simply about maintaining energy during a ride, but also effective recovery after, so that you can gear up and roll out for your next cycling adventure with gusto. The power is quite literally in your hands—and your snack pack!

Chapter 5. Choosing the Right Energy Snacks: A Comprehensive Analysis

Before we delve into specific energy snacks, it's crucial to understand why nutrition plays a pivotal role in cycling performance. Cycling, whether recreational or professional, places significant stress on the body. To maintain energy levels and ensure optimal performance, cyclists need to fuel their bodies aptly.

The science behind this concept rests on the pivotal roles of carbohydrates, proteins, and fats in energy metabolism. Carbohydrates are the body's preferred source of energy during intense activity, while protein assists with muscle repair and recovery. Although fats are a dense energy source, the body uses them more readily during lower-intensity, endurance-based activities.

Let's delve into choosing the right energy snacks for your ride.

5.1. In-Ride Nutrition Strategies and Choices

An optimal in-ride nutrition strategy encompasses hydration, macro and micronutrients. These factors all contribute to maintaining energy levels, reducing muscle tissue breakdown, and sustaining hydration.

1. Hydration — Alongside nutrient intake, hydration is absolutely crucial. Dehydration can affect aerobic capacity, reduce blood volume, and lead to overheating. Electrolyte sports drinks are recommended as they contain sodium and potassium that help

maintain fluid balance.

2. Carbohydrates — During intense cycling, the body relies heavily on carbs as an immediate energy source. Energy gels, bananas, and sports drinks are excellent sources of quick-release carbs.

3. Protein — Although rides don't typically require protein intake, for longer rides, eating a small amount of protein-rich snacks like a protein bar or nuts can help minimize tissue breakdown.

4. Fats — During longer, less intense rides, healthy fats, such as nuts or avocados, can provide sustainable energy.

5.2. The Power of Portable and Convenient Snacks

A crucial aspect when choosing cycling snacks is convenience. These should be portable, easy to open/eat while cycling, and not spoil in outdoor conditions.

1. Energy Bars: They are nutrient-dense, available in a variety of flavors, and specifically formulated to provide a balance of carbs, protein, and fats.

2. Energy Gels: Offering a concentrated source of quick-release energy, gels can give you an immediate energy boost during a ride.

3. Nut Butter: Single-serving packets of nut butter, preferably almond or peanut, are packed with protein and healthy fats, offering sustained energy.

4. Dried Fruits and Nuts: Lightweight and easy to pack, dried fruits give you a natural sugar kick, while nuts provide protein and fats.

5.3. Timing Your Snack Intake For Optimal Performance

Timing your energy intake is vital for maintaining energy levels during your ride. As a general rule, aim to consume a snack every 45-60 minutes during a long ride. But, remember that everyone's needs differ, so it's essential to find what works best for you.

5.4. Refuelling Post-Ride: The Importance of Recovery Snacks

Adequate recovery nutrition after a cycling session speeds up muscle tissue repair and replenishes energy reserves. This includes a balance of protein and carbs; protein for muscle repair and carbs for replacing glycogen stores. Snacks like a protein shake with fruits or a yogurt parfait with granola, fruit, and nuts can be a great post-ride choice.

These nutritional strategies can significantly enhance your cycling performance, helping you feel energized and productive throughout your rides. Uncover your optimal fuel strategy and elevate your cycling experience to a whole new level.

Chapter 6. Pre-Ride Nutrition: Fueling Up for the Journey

Starting your cycling journey on the right foot - or rather, the right bite - can be the pivotal factor that determines the performance and enjoyment of your ride. Nutrition plays a vital role in your cycling performance, not just during the ride but significantly, beforehand. This chapter intricately explores the science of pre-ride fueling, providing practical strategies and exhibiting the transformative power of well-timed nutrition.

6.1. The Foundation of Pre-Ride Nutrition

Understanding the basics of nutrition is imperative to optimize your energy levels for cycling. Our bodies utilize different nutrients for various functions. For strenuous physical activities such as cycling, the primary source of fuel is carbohydrates, which are stored in the body as glycogen.

Ideally, you should aim to start your ride with high glycogen stores, which you achieve by consuming a carbohydrate-rich meal a few hours before you get on the bike. This gives your body time to digest and convert the food into fuel. Alongside carbohydrates, proteins and fats should form a part of your pre-ride meal, albeit in lesser quantities.

Your hydration status is equally essential. Start your ride well-hydrated by consuming fluids (water or sports drinks) in the hours leading up to your cycling session.

6.2. Building Your Pre-Ride Meal

Creating the perfect pre-ride meal combines the science of nutrition with individual preferences. The aim is to consume a meal rich in carbohydrates, moderate in protein, low in fat and fiber, and packed with fluids.

1. Carbohydrates: They are your body's preferred form of quick energy. Sources can include whole-grain bread, cereals, pasta, rice, fruits, and energy bars.

2. Proteins: Necessary for repair and recovery, protein sources could include lean meats, yogurt, milk, or a protein shake.

3. Fats: Healthy fats should be incorporated but in minimum amounts as they slow digestion. Avocados, nuts, and seeds are good options.

4. Fluids: Hydrate with water, sports drinks, or even herbal teas.

Remember that the size and timing of your pre-ride meal varies according to your ride length and intensity. For a long and intense ride, a larger meal consumed 3-4 hours before can be beneficial. For shorter rides, a light meal or snack even 1-2 hours beforehand may suffice.

6.3. Listening to Your Body: Personalizing Your Meal Plan

Nutrition is not a one-size-fits-all solution. Each cyclist needs to understand his or her body's responses and adjust accordingly. Keep in mind these key considerations while customizing your intake:

1. Gastrointestinal comfort: Monitor how your body reacts to different foods and identify any that cause discomfort.

2. Timing: Pay attention to how different timings affect your energy

levels. This is a process of trial and error.

3. Size and satiety: Do not overeat. The goal is to feel satisfied, not stuffed.

6.4. Supplements: Are They Necessary?

Thoughtfully chosen nutritional supplements may provide performance benefits. However, they should be considered as additions to an already balanced diet, and not substitutes for whole foods. Potential useful supplements can include caffeine, beetroot juice, or beta-alanine.

6.5. Bottom Line

Pre-ride nutrition, when done well, not only increases your chances of a stellar cycling session but also aids your overall health. It seems like a complex balancing act, but it becomes second nature with understanding, experimentation, and consistency.

Your cycling journey is not just about the path traveled but also the fuel that powers your ride. By arming yourself with knowledge and applying it sensibly, you set yourself up for a ride that's not just endurable, but enjoyable. Tasting the sweet success of your cycling goals begins with the first bite of your pre-ride meal. Happy fueling and happy cycling!

Chapter 7. During-Ride Snacking: Maintaining Your Energy Levels

There's no denying the fundamental role of on-the-bike nutrition in optimizing cycling performance. Whether you're popping out for a quick spin or attempting a challenging climb, what you consume during your ride can certainly make the difference between failure and success. The balance of hydration, carbohydrate, electrolyte, and even protein intake can impact your overall energy levels, cognitive function, and muscle performance.

7.1. Hydration: A Balance Between Thirst and Requirement

Getting hydration right is the first step when it comes to in-ride snacking. Dehydration can be a performance killer, leading to early fatigue, reduced endurance, and mental fog. So, how much fluid should you be consuming? To maintain optimal hydration levels, aim to drink around 500ml-1000ml (16.9oz-33.8oz) of an electrolyte drink per hour, depending on factors such as intensity, temperature, and individual sweat rates.

Water forms the base of your hydration strategy. When cycling at low intensities for less than 60 minutes in cool conditions, plain water often suffices. However, when the intensity cranks up or the ride extends beyond the 60-minute mark, adding electrolytes and carbohydrates becomes crucial. Electrolytes, particularly sodium, aid in fluid retention and reduce the diuretic effect of excessive water consumption. Meanwhile, adding carbohydrates assists with energy provision and enhances fluid absorption in the gut.

7.2. Carbohydrates: Fuelling your Muscles

Your muscles primarily run on glycogen – a stored form of carbohydrate in the muscles and liver. For rides longer than 90 minutes, getting enough carbohydrates becomes crucial as your body starts to deplete its glycogen stores.

If carbohydrate intake doesn't match the expenditure, performance decreases and fatigue sets in. Therefore, to prevent "bonking" or "hitting the wall," aim for 30-60 grams of carbohydrate per hour of exercise. This will maintain blood sugar levels and spare muscle glycogen stores for later during the trip.

There are many options available for in-ride carbs. Energy gels, chews, and bars are all effective sources. For those who prefer whole foods, bananas, dates, and rice cakes are excellent options.

Remember that the idea is to gradually feed your body with carbs. Tests have shown that a steady influx of carbs usually results in better performance than getting the same amount in fewer, larger doses. So, instead of downing an energy gel all at once, take small bites or sips every 15 minutes.

7.3. Fuelling the Mind: Glucose - a Brain Booster?

While providing energy for your muscles, carbohydrates also play a pivotal role in maintaining focus and decision-making ability during the ride. Glucose literally fuels the brain, helping to keep mental fatigue at bay. So, don't undervalue the cognitive benefit of regular carb intake during your rides.

7.4. Protein: Is it Necessary During the Ride?

The verdict is still out on protein consumption during the ride. While it's typically not regarded as immediately necessary, there is emerging research indicating that consuming small amounts of protein alongside carbohydrates may reduce muscle damage and improve overall performance during longer, more strenuous rides.

Protein-based energy bars or drinks might make an excellent choice for those venturing out on extensive multi-hour rides or multi-day cycle tours where muscle damage and recovery become more critical.

7.5. When and How to Eat On the Bike

As a rule of thumb, start eating before you feel hungry. The onset of hunger often means your glucose levels are already too low. Begin sipping your carbohydrate drink or eating your selected snacks 30-45 minutes into your ride. From there on, aim to get a little something every 15-20 minutes.

Cycling nutrition technique also matters. When eating gels, bars, or bites, do not swallow them in one gulp. Instead, take small bites and let them dissolve in your mouth. This maximizes carbohydrate absorption and minimizes the risk of digestive discomfort.

Remember to test different options during your training rides to find the snacks and hydration mixtures that best suit your stomach and taste preference.

7.6. Bib Shorts with Pockets – A Key Snack Storage Tip

To make your snacking more manageable, bib shorts with pockets can be a game-changer. These pockets can house your gels, bars, or total food intake for the ride. It saves you from reaching into your jersey pocket every time, thus offering constant and easy access to your nutrition.

A well-planned in-ride snacking strategy, combined with training and recovery, can make a substantial difference in your cycling performance. By keeping these facts in mind, finding the best during-ride eating strategy that works for you can be a game-changer for your cycling adventures. So, fuel up and enjoy the ride!

Chapter 8. Post-Ride Recovery: Refueling After Your Journey

Replenishing essential nutrients is critical post-ride, as it aids the body in its fundamental recovery processes. Cyclists who practice strategic refueling optimize muscle repair, bolster immunity, and prepare themselves for future sprints, hills, and high-intensity efforts.

8.1. Understanding the Importance of Refueling

At the end of a ride, your muscles are in a state of breakdown from strenuous exertion. They have, in effect, depleted their glycogen stores (your body's prime source of energy during moderate to high-intensity cycling) and have sustained microscopic damage. They are crying out for replenishment and repair, ideally within a short window of opportunity meeting often referred to as the 'golden hour'.

The 'golden hour', typically the first 30 to 60 minutes after exercise, is when your muscles are most receptive to nutrients. Consuming the right combination of nutrients during this window kickstarts your recovery immediately, promoting a swift return to full strength and potentially enhancing your overall cycling performance.

8.2. Nutrient Composition: Protein, Carbohydrates, and Fats

Refueling isn't simply about eating as soon as possible after your ride. It's important to ingest the right types of food in the appropriate proportions.

Proteins: Consuming ample protein–ideally around 20 grams–directly following a workout is critical because these amino acid-rich foods provide the raw material for muscle repair and new muscle growth.

Carbohydrates: Because your body primarily uses stored glycogen as fuel for high-intensity exercise like cycling, it's crucial to replenish these reserves. Consuming carbohydrates soon after your ride helps restore glycogen stores more effectively.

Fats: Don't shy away from fats post-exercise! While it may seem counterintuitive after burning so many calories, some intake of healthy fats enables efficient absorption of nutrients and helps manage inflammation.

8.3. Hydration: Replacing Lost Fluids

Hydration should never be an afterthought—it's just as important, if not more so, than eating post-ride. While cycling, your body loses fluids and electrolytes through sweating. These losses can result in dehydration if not properly addressed. Even minor dehydration could lead to significant reductions in performance and recovery.

An ideal hydration strategy post-riding is to consume 150% of the weight loss over the four to six hours post-ride. For example, if you have lost a kilogram during your ride, aim to consume 1.5 liters of fluid over the next few hours.

8.4. Recovery Foods and Snacks

Post-ride, meals and snacks should be rich in protein and carbohydrates. Aim to consume between a 3:1 and 4:1 ratio of carbs to protein–this can expedite glycogen storage and muscle repair.

Excellent post-ride meals include lean protein and complex carbs, such as chicken breast, salmon, whole grain bread, and quinoa. Snacks like Greek yogurt, a protein shake, or a carbohydrate-rich fruit like bananas are worth considering.

8.5. Recover and Become Stronger

After a hard ride, it may be tempting to kick back and relax, but don't neglect your nutrition! The 'golden hour' post-ride is a critical window during which the right nutrients can really boost your recovery and overall strength. Always ensure a strategic blend of protein, carbohydrates, and healthy fats post-ride and pay close attention to hydration. With the right post-ride regimen, you're not just bouncing back–you're becoming a stronger, more efficient cyclist.

The journey to optimizing your nutrition and performance on the saddle does not end here. Keep exploring, experimenting, and tuning your strategy to find what works best for your body. Happy riding!

Chapter 9. Food vs. Supplements: The Perks and Pitfalls

Food and supplements both play a critical role when it comes to fueling your body for cycling. Your goal should be to find a balance between the two, understanding when to fuel with whole foods and when to opt for supplements. To help you manage this balancing act, we'll look at the perks and pitfalls of each.

9.1. Whole Foods: The All-Natural Fuel Source

Whole foods are nutritionally dense and supply a combination of carbohydrates, fats, proteins, and other necessary nutrients for optimal body functioning and energy production. Consuming a variety of whole foods ensures you obtain an array of vitamins, minerals, and other beneficial compounds, many of which are not available in supplements.

They also provide fiber, which promotes digestive health and helps with satiety, potentially making you feel fuller for longer periods. This can be especially useful during longer rides. But remember, eating whole foods close to your ride could cause discomfort, so it's essential to time it right. A balanced meal 2-3 hours before exercising is advisable.

9.2. The Downside of Whole Foods During Rides

Unfortunately, whole foods can be inconvenient to transport and consume during a ride. They often require preparation and storage, which isn't always practical during cycling. Additionally, consuming whole foods while performing vigorous activity can sometimes lead to digestive discomfort.

9.3. Energy Supplements: Quick and Convenient

Energy supplements, which come in various forms - energy bars, gels, chews, and sports drinks, are designed to rapidly deliver nutrients to your body. They come pre-packaged and are easily transported and consumed, making them particularly useful during a ride.

Most of these rations provide a high amount of carbohydrates, the body's preferred energy source during high-intensity activities such as cycling. Some supplements deliver fast-acting sugars for immediate energy, whilst others provide complex carbohydrates for sustained release.

9.4. Risks and Limitations of Supplements

While supplements can be beneficial, they do come with pitfalls. They are not designed to replace whole foods, only to be consumed around exercise for a timely energy jolt. Over-relying on supplements could lead to nutrient deficiencies as they do not provide all the essential nutrients your body requires for overall health.

In addition to nutrient deficiencies, an excessive consumption of energy supplements can lead to gastrointestinal distress due to the high sugar content and artificial ingredients present in some products. Each individual tolerates supplements differently, so it's advisable to test various products during training before using them in a race or longer ride.

9.5. The Balance: Combining Food and Supplements

Achieving balance between whole foods and energy supplements will depend on factors such as the duration and intensity of your cycle, your personal nutritional needs, and your tastebuds. A practical approach might be to rely on whole foods for daily nutrition and endurance training, using energy supplements before and during high-intensity workouts or races for added energy.

9.6. Develop Your Personal Fueling Plan

Understanding your own nutritional needs is an essential step in crafting your perfect balance between food and supplements. Factors like your age, sex, weight, fitness level, and cycling goals will all influence your nutritional requirements.

Consider visiting a sports dietitian or nutritionist who specializes in endurance sports. They can provide personalized advice and guidance, helping you to create an individual food and supplement plan that is designed to support your cycling ambitions.

Our bodies are different, what works for one individual may not work for another. Embrace the process of finding out what best fuels your journey and enjoy the ride!

9.7. Conclusion

Whole foods and supplements both have their place in a cyclist's diet.

Whole foods provide a complete nutritional profile, while supplements offer convenience and quick energy, especially during on-the-move scenarios. Striking the right balance can boost your cycling performance while also ensuring you're meeting all your essential nutritional needs.

Remember, food vs. supplements isn't an either-or scenario, but rather a delicate balance where both elements work together to fuel your two-wheeled adventures. The key is to understand your personal nutritional needs and how to align these with your cycling goals. This careful calibration allows you to reach your peak performance, optimizing energy, recovery, and overall well-being.

Now, it's time to roll and take your ride to the next level with a right fuel mix of whole foods and supplements. Enjoy the journey!

Note: Always consult a healthcare professional before making any changes to your diet or taking new dietary supplements.

Chapter 10. Hydration and Cycling: The Role of Fluids and Electrolytes

Cycling, regardless of its intensity, demands an unmatched level of physical exertion. One of the most critical components to help sustain this effort is proper hydration. Our bodies, made up of around 60% of water, need to maintain adequate fluid levels to function optimally. Ensuring correct hydration and electrolyte balance can drastically improve your cycling performance and overall experience.

10.1. Understanding the Importance of Hydration

Stay tuned with your water intake, because even mild dehydration can considerably hinder your performance. When the body's water content drops, it leads to decreased blood volume, which in turn makes the heart work harder to push out the essential nutrients, oxygen, and ATP (adenosine triphosphate) to the working muscles. Not just that, but dehydration can also reduce cognitive function, impair judgement and coordination — certainly not an ideal situation when on a bike!

Water also plays a vital role in cooling down the body, especially during intensive cycling sessions. Your body tends to overheat when working out. To regulate the body temperature, sweat glands excrete water which evaporates from the skin's surface, thereby providing a cooling effect. But remember — sweat isn't just water but also consists of critical electrolytes that need to be replaced.

10.2. Electrolytes: The Tiny Powerhouses

Electrolytes, the tiny powerhouses, are minerals that carry an electric charge within the body. Sodium, potassium, calcium, magnesium, and chloride are some of the primary electrolytes essential for the body. These play crucial roles in maintaining fluid and acid-base balance, muscle contractions, neural activity, blood clotting, and more.

Imagine cycling up an incline—it's demanding, right? It would require substantial muscle contractions, which, as you may have guessed, are governed by these electrolytes. Lower levels of electrolytes, also known as electrolyte imbalance, can impede your cycling performance. Electrolyte imbalance can lead to fatigue, cramping, and in severe cases, it can induce life-threatening conditions like hyponatremia (low sodium) or hyperkalemia (high potassium).

10.3. Gauging Hydration Levels: Understanding Thirst

While thirst might seem like the logical flag for when you need to drink, it isn't always the most reliable indicator, especially when you're engaged in strenuous physical exercise like cycling. In such circumstances, your body is likely to be dehydrated to some degree before you even start to feel thirsty. Therefore, understanding the colour of your urine can serve as a better indicator of your hydration status. Light-coloured or clear urine suggests that you're well hydrated, whereas darker urine often points towards dehydration.

10.4. Hydration Strategies for Cycling

Cycling requires strategic hydration. Start hydrating the night before a big ride or a race, focusing especially on balancing your electrolyte levels. Try to consume at least 500 ml (about 17 ounces) of fluids two hours before setting off.

During your ride, aim for approximately 500 to 1000 ml (17 to 34 ounces) of hydration for each hour, depending on your physical attributes, intensity of the ride, and the weather conditions. Hydrating every 15 to 20 minutes with small quantities can be more conducive than gulping huge amounts infrequently. This helps your body better absorb the fluids rather than quickly passing right through you.

It's all about maintaining a balance. Drinking too much water without adequate electrolyte replacement can lead to hyponatremia. And on the other hand, excessive consumption of electrolytes can result in hyperkalemia.

10.5. Post-Ride Hydration and Recovery

Post-ride hydration and recovery are just as essential as maintaining hydration during the ride. Your post-cycling regime should focus on replenishing the fluid and electrolyte losses incurred during your ride. Rehydration helps kick-start the recovery process, rebuild damaged muscle tissues, and refill the energy stores in your body.

A general rule of thumb is to consume 1.5 times the volume of fluid lost during the exercise. But how can you determine the volume lost? Weigh yourself before and after your ride. Each kilogram lost translates to approximately one litre of fluid that needs to be replaced.

For balanced hydration, opt for fluids containing sodium, as sodium will not only help retain water but also stimulate your thirst, encouraging you to drink more. Try to avoid alcoholic beverages post-ride, as these can accelerate dehydration.

So, whether you're soaring over steep mountain trails or skimming through the bustling city streets, precise hydration and understanding how electrolytes work can make a significant difference in your cycling performance as well as recovery. Equip yourself with this vital knowledge, and make each ride a successful journey.

Chapter 11. Personalizing Your Cycling Nutrition: Tailoring Your Fuel to Your Needs

Understanding the impact of nutrition on your cycling performance and overall health is a journey. And, like any journey, it's not one-size-fits-all. Bodies vary, so do their energy needs and the ways they process different types of fuel. This section aims to guide you through the process of personalizing your cycling nutrition, tailoring your fuel intake to your individual needs. We'll cover the determining factors for your personal nutritional requirements, offer strategies to translate these into a functional cycling diet, and provide guidance on adjusting your nutrition plan in line with your changing needs and goals.

11.1. Riding: Demanding Different Fuels

Knowing what to eat and when, starts with the understanding that different types of riding require different types of fuel. Three crucial factors for determining the best fuel to power your ride are: Duration, Intensity, and Frequency of your rides.

Long-duration, low-intensity rides, such as endurance training rides, generally require a higher proportion of fat for fuel. On the other hand, shorter, high-intensity rides, like sprints or climbs, rely more on carbohydrates. If you're riding multiple times a day or training for a high-frequency event, protein becomes more important for muscle repair and growth.

Start by analyzing your riding pattern. Note down the typical duration, intensity, and frequency of your rides. This will help in customizing your nutrition plan.

11.2. Body Size, Composition, and Metabolism

Your body's size, fat to muscle ratio, and metabolic efficiency also play substantial roles in determining your individual nutritional needs. A larger body requires more fuel intake, whereas a body with more muscle burns energy more rapidly and therefore, necessitates more protein for repair and growth. Lastly, someone with a fast metabolism will go through fuel more quickly than someone whose metabolism is relatively slow.

To establish your specific nutritional needs, you may need to consult a healthcare or fitness professional for body composition and metabolic rate testing. This, coupled with a clear understanding of your riding habits, will form the basis of your personalized nutritional plan.

11.3. Assessing Need vs Intake

Having established your needs, the next step is to assess your current nutritional intake. You can track what you eat in a week, noting everything from meals to beverages, energy bars, and any additional snacks. This will provide you a clearer picture of your existing calorie and nutrient consumption.

Use this data to calculate your daily averages of caloric intake, fat, protein, and carbohydrate consumption. This will act as your starting point for tailoring your dietary practices to your unique needs and objectives.

11.4. Crafting a Personalized Nutrition Plan

Now that you have a clear view of both your nutrition needs and your current intake, you can start formulating your personalized nutrition plan.

If, for example, you found that your current energy intake is lower than what's needed for your riding schedule and body metabolism, you would need to increase your intake. On the other hand, if you're consuming unnecessary excess calories, you'll need to moderate your food intake or redistribute your intake for more efficiency.

Remember, your body fuels its cycling using both carbohydrates and fats, and muscle maintenance and repair require protein. Ensure that any revisions to your nutrition plan take this into account. Aim to achieve a dynamic balance between these macronutrients, and consider the timing of your intake to optimize your body's fuel efficiency.

11.5. Reacting to Body Feedback and Monitoring Changes

Food and nutrient intake should not only be about feeding the ride. Digestive comfort, overall health, and well-being, as well as maintaining a joy for eating, should also be taken into consideration. Listen to your body's responses. If certain foods or eating schedules cause discomfort, review and adjust your plan accordingly.

To monitor the effectiveness of your tailored diet plan, track changes in your riding performance and overall health. Remember, it's crucial to remain flexible and willing to alter your plan as necessary. As you adapt, your diet plan will likely need to adapt with you.

11.6. Wrapping Up

Creating a personalized nutrition and fueling plan for cycling can significantly enhance your performance, recovery, and overall experience on and off the bike. Start your journey into personalized cycling nutrition today, and witness the positive impact of strength fueled by understanding and strategy.

Remember, every ride and every body is different. Embrace the differences and use them to your advantage. The flexibility and power that comes with knowing your body and what it needs will make you an unstoppable force on your bike. Engineer your eating to optimize your energy, and let the wheels roll towards your new healthier, high-performing cycling adventure.